Lupus Awareness

Bridging Understanding, Inspiring Change

Rossana Lewis

TABLE OF CONTENT

Chapter 1: Understanding Lupus

1.1 What is Lupus?

Lupus is a disease that occurs when your body's immune system attacks your own tissues and organs (autoimmune disease). Inflammation caused by lupus can affect many different body systems, including your joints, skin, kidneys, blood cells, brain, heart and lungs.

Lupus can be difficult to diagnose because its signs and symptoms often mimic those of other ailments. The most distinctive sign of lupus — a facial rash that resembles the wings of a butterfly unfolding across both cheeks — occurs in many but not all cases of lupus.

Some people are born with a tendency toward developing lupus, which may be triggered by infections, certain drugs or even sunlight. While there's no cure for lupus, treatments can help control symptoms.

1.2 Types of Lupus

Healthcare providers sometimes call lupus systemic lupus erythematosus (SLE). It's the most common type of lupus, and means you have lupus throughout your body. Other types include:

Cutaneous Lupus Erythematosus: Lupus that only affects your skin.

Drug-Induced Lupus: Some medications trigger lupus symptoms as a side effect. It's usually temporary and might go away after you stop taking the medication that caused it.

Neonatal Lupus: Babies are sometimes born with lupus. Babies born to biological parents with lupus aren't certain to have lupus, but they might have an increased risk.

1.3 Causes and Triggers

Causes

Experts don't know for certain what causes lupus. Studies have found that certain factors about your health or where you live may trigger lupus:

Genetic Factors: Having certain genetic mutations may make you more likely to have lupus.

Hormones: Reactions to certain hormones in your body (especially estrogen) may make you more likely to develop lupus.

Environmental Factors: Aspects about where you live and how much pollution or sunlight you're exposed to might affect your lupus risk.

Health History: Smoking, your stress level and having certain other health conditions (like other autoimmune diseases) might trigger lupus.

Triggers

Lupus is known for its unpredictable nature, often characterized by periods of remission and flare-ups. Identifying triggers that can exacerbate symptoms is crucial in managing the condition effectively:

Sunlight and UV Exposure: Exposure to sunlight or artificial ultraviolet light can trigger skin rashes, known as photosensitivity, and worsen Lupus symptoms.

Stress: Emotional stress and physical stressors can potentially trigger Lupus flares or exacerbate existing symptoms. Stress management techniques are essential for individuals living with Lupus.

Infections: Certain infections, such as viral or bacterial infections, can prompt Lupus flares. Managing and promptly treating infections is crucial in minimizing their impact on Lupus symptoms.

Medications: Some medications, particularly antibiotics, blood pressure drugs, and anti-seizure medications, may trigger Lupus flares in susceptible individuals. Discussing medication management with a healthcare professional is crucial.

Hormonal Changes: Hormonal fluctuations, such as those occurring during pregnancy, menstruation, or menopause, can influence Lupus symptoms in some individuals.

Risk Factors

Anyone can develop lupus, but some groups of people have a higher risk:

- People assigned female at birth (AFAB), especially people AFAB between the ages of 15 and 44.
- Black people.
- Hispanic people.
- Asian people.

- Native Americans, Alaska Natives and First Nations people.
- Pacific Islanders.
- People with a biological parent who has lupus.

Chapter 2: Signs and Symptoms

2.1 Common Symptoms of Lupus

Lupus causes symptoms throughout your body, depending on which organs or systems it affects. Everyone experiences a different combination and severity of symptoms.

Lupus symptoms usually come and go in waves called flare-ups. During a flare-up, the symptoms can be severe enough to affect your daily routine. You might also have periods of remission when you have mild or no symptoms.

Symptoms usually develop slowly. You might notice one or two signs of lupus at first, and then more or different symptoms later on. The most common symptoms include:

- Joint pain, muscle pain or chest pain (especially when you're taking a deep breath).
- Headaches.
- Rashes (it's common to have a rash across your face that providers sometimes call a butterfly rash).
- Fever.
- Hair loss.
- Mouth sores.
- Fatigue (feeling tired all the time).
- Shortness of breath (dyspnea).
- Swollen glands.
- Swelling in your arms, legs or on your face.
- Confusion.
- Blood clots.

Lupus can sometimes cause other health conditions or issues, including:

- Photosensitivity (sensitivity to sunlight).
- Dry eye.
- Depression (or other mental health conditions).
- Seizures.
- Anemia.
- Raynaud's syndrome.
- Osteoporosis.
- Heart disease.
- Kidney disease.

2.2 Diagnosis and Tests

A healthcare provider will diagnose lupus with a physical exam and some tests. They'll examine your symptoms and talk to you about what you're experiencing. Tell your provider when you first noticed symptoms or changes in your body. Your provider will ask about your medical history, including conditions you may have now and how you're treating or managing them.

Lupus can be tricky to diagnose because it can affect so many parts of your body and cause lots of different symptoms. Even small changes or issues that seem unusual for you can be a key. Don't be afraid to tell your provider about anything you've felt or sensed — you know your body better than anyone.

There's not one test that can confirm a lupus diagnosis. Diagnosing it is usually part of a differential diagnosis. This means your provider will probably use a few tests to determine what's causing your symptoms before ruling out other conditions and diagnosing you with lupus. They might use:

- Blood tests to see how well your immune system is working and to check for infections or other issues like anemia or low blood cell counts.

- Urinalysis to check your pee for signs of infections or other health conditions.

- An antinuclear antibody (ANA) test looks for antibodies (protein markers that show a history of your body fighting off infections). People who have lupus usually have certain antibodies that show their immune system has been overly active.

- A biopsy of your skin or kidney tissue can show if your immune system has damaged them.

2.3 Recognizing Flares

A lupus flare is a temporary period of time when your particular lupus symptoms feel worse in a way your provider can measure (by examining you or with a lab test). It often requires a change in treatment.

Lupus flares are different for each person, since everyone has their own version of lupus. When your lupus flares, the symptoms of your lupus will be worse than normal. Sometimes, new symptoms can also occur.

For example, let's say you get rashes and joint pain when your lupus is not well controlled. During a lupus flare, you could expect to have rashes, joint pain, and possibly a new symptom, too.

Some common symptoms of lupus flares include:

- Painful and swollen joints
- Rashes
- Sores in the mouth or nose
- Fatigue
- Fevers (not caused by infection)
- Abnormal blood or urine test results

Chapter 3: Managing Lupus

3.1 Medications and Treatments

Your healthcare provider will suggest treatments for lupus that manage your symptoms. The goal is minimizing damage to your organs and how much lupus affects your day-to-day life. Most people with lupus need a combination of medications to help them prevent flare-ups and lessen their symptom severity during one. You might need:

Hydroxychloroquine: Hydroxychloroquine is a prescription antiviral medication that can relieve lupus symptoms and slow down how they progress (change or get worse).

Nonsteroidal Anti-Inflammatory Drugs (NSAIDs): Over-the-counter (OTC) NSAIDs relieve pain and reduce inflammation. Your provider will tell you which type of NSAID will work best for you, and how often you should take it. Don't take NSAIDs for more than 10 days in a row without talking to your provider.

Corticosteroids: Corticosteroids are prescription medications that reduce inflammation. Prednisone is a common corticosteroid providers use to manage lupus. Your provider might prescribe you pills you take by mouth or inject a corticosteroid directly into one of your joints.

Immunosuppressants: Immunosuppressants are medications that hold back your immune system and stop it from being as active. They can help prevent tissue damage and inflammation.

3.2 Lifestyle Changes for Managing Symptoms

Lifestyle changes can't cure lupus but they can help handle symptoms, improve quality of life, and lower the risk of problems from it. You will also need to find a balance for your physical and mental health.

Quit Smoking: Smoking alters each cell in the body. It also causes stress on the heart, lungs, and kidneys. The stress can worsen lupus. Quitting will have good benefits on your health right away. If you smoke, talk to your doctor about how you can quit.

Avoid Being in the Sun: Lupus makes many people more likely to get a sunburn. Sunlight can also worsen its skin rashes and cause it to flare up. To protect yourself:

- Avoid the sun, chiefly between 10 am and 4 pm.
- Wear sunscreen with at least 30 SPF.
- Wear a hat, long sleeves, and clothing that covers all of your legs.

Avoiding Infection: Lupus and some of the drugs used to treat it also lower the immune system. This puts you at a higher risk of infections. Infections may come more often or last longer. To protect yourself:

- Make sure you are up to date and have gotten all your vaccines.
- Get the yearly flu shot.
- Get the pneumococcal shot.
- Do not be around people who are sick, even if it is just a common cold.

- Wash your hands often, especially after being in contact with someone who is sick.

Not all infections can be stopped. Get care right away if you think you have one.

Diet: A healthy diet is vital for your well-being. Be sure to get enough fruits, veggies, and whole grains. Dietary changes may also be needed if you have things like high blood pressure, kidney disease, or digestive problems. Omega-3 fatty acids may help lower lupus activity. Omega-3 is found in fatty fish and certain plant seed oils. It is also available in supplement form, but it is best to get it from foods.

It may be helpful to avoid alfalfa, but there are no other foods that start flare-ups. Keep a food diary. Do not eat foods that make your symptoms worse.

Also, limit alcohol as it can affect how medicines work or worsen problems that you may have. Moderation is two drinks per day for men and one drink per day for women.

Lower Stress: Stress can put an extra burden on your body. It can also weaken your immune system and worsen symptoms. Look for ways to reduce it, such as lifestyle changes or meditation. It can be stressful to manage lupus. Consider joining a support group. If you have a hard time getting out, consider using video chat, email, or social networking. Try not to isolate yourself. Stay in touch with your friends.

Exercise: Exercise can help with your strength and well-being. This can lessen the effects of lupus. Activities may need to be adjusted during flare ups, but complete bed rest is rarely helpful. Talk with your doctor before you start an exercise program. Exercise programs can focus on avoiding problem areas, such as a sore hip. An exercise physiologist or physical therapist can help design a safe and helpful program.

Avoid Depression: It is common to feel mood changes, especially within the first few months of a new diagnosis or during a flare up. Depression can slow your recovery and put you at risk for more serious health problems.
Call your doctor if you have feelings of sadness, hopelessness, and loss of interest in activities that last for two weeks. There are several

treatment options available, such as counseling and medicines.

Returning to Everyday Life:

- Take an Active Role in Your Care: Keep in touch with your medical team. Let them know if you are having signs that a flare up may be coming. Talk to them about symptoms or treatments that you are having a hard time with. There may be other treatment options to help you manage your health.

- Sex: It is normal for you or your partner to feel worried about sexual activity. Lupus impacts sex and your relationship. You and your partner may be referred to individual or couples therapy. It will help you both talk about your concerns.

- Counseling: Support groups or one-on-one counseling can help you cope with challenges. Support groups let you talk with others who have experiences like yours. They offer a setting of encouragement and support that will help you adjust and stick to your treatment.

3.3 Coping with Emotional Challenges

Living with lupus can have a profound effect on a person's mental and emotional well-being. You may have recently been diagnosed with lupus, or you may have been living with it for years. Either way, you are likely to have experienced mental and physical problems such as difficulty concentrating or sleeping. You are also likely to have felt emotions such as grief, fear, anxiety, and depression. These feelings are common.

There are steps you can take to cope better with lupus, including:

Educating Yourself and Others: Learn as much as you can about the disease and its treatment. Share information with friends and family members so they will better understand the disease and how it affects you. Their support is important to success in managing the illness.

Practicing Healthy Lifestyle Habits: Exercise regularly; eat a healthy, balanced diet; get enough rest; and avoid alcoholic beverages, particularly if you are depressed. Alcohol is a natural depressant. It can markedly increase the severity of depression and its symptoms.

Learning Stress-Management Techniques: Living with a chronic disease is stressful. A mental health professional can teach you techniques, such as progressive muscle relaxation, guided imagery, and meditation, that you can use regularly to cope with the stress of lupus. Other stress relievers you can try include listening to soothing music, taking a warm bath or a walk, or doing some gentle exercises.

Doing Activities you Enjoy: Lupus may limit some activities. So it's important to find things you enjoy doing and take time to do them. These activities can be as simple as reading a good book or doing thoughtful things for others.

Seeking Support: When you are feeling down, talk with a trusted friend, clergy member, or counselor. Consider joining a support group. To find a group for lupus patients near you, speak with your doctor or counselor or check with the

Arthritis Foundation or Lupus Foundation of America.

Appreciating Yourself: Although you have lupus, you likely have many other things, such as pretty eyes, a friendly smile, musical talent, or a flare for Cajun cooking. Don't make lupus the focus of your life. Focus on your talents, abilities, and strengths.

Chapter 4: Living Well with Lupus

4.1 Diet and Nutrition

There is no food that can cure lupus. Lupus is an autoimmune disease, an illness that can affect many body systems. The foods that you eat, however, and the medications you take may have an effect on some of your symptoms. It is also important to understand that there is a link between lupus and osteoporosis and cardiovascular disease. Healthy nutrition can greatly affect those with these co-occurring diseases. Nutrition may impact the symptoms and outcomes of these co-occurring illnesses.

How Does Food Affect Those with Lupus?

A well-balanced diet with proper nutrition can positively benefit those living with lupus in the following ways:

- Reduce inflammation (redness and swelling) and other symptoms
- Prevent nutrient deficiencies
- Maintain strong bones and muscle
- Combat side-effects of medications
- Achieve or maintain desirable weight
- Reduce risk of heart disease

What Foods Should be a Part of Your Diet?

There are some important general nutrition guidelines for individuals with lupus. Some key guidelines include diets low in fat, cholesterol, and sodium; low in refined sugars like soda and concentrated juices; and high in fiber. It is important to be aware of high protein diets which can often stress the kidneys. Most importantly, it is imperative to keep a well-balanced diet.

There are some key foods that are important for your diet. Having a balance is essential – that is, to not eat too much of one thing and not enough of another. Different foods have different nutritional components. Try to include a variety of fruits and vegetables; foods low in calories and saturated fats; and foods high in antioxidants, fiber, calcium, vitamin D, and Omega 3 fatty acids.

Fruits and Vegetables: Fruits and vegetables contain antioxidants and fiber. They are a great source of Vitamin A and Vitamin C. Some healthy ways to add fruits and vegetables into your diet:

- Snack on fruits and vegetables throughout the day
- Add vegetables to soups, sandwiches, and salads
- Add vegetables to all of your meals
- Add fruit to make smoothies
- Add fruit to your cereal and yogurt
- Choose fresh and/or frozen (without sauces)
- Go easy on canned foods (choose low salt), dried fruits, and fruit juice

Healthy Fats and Oils: Not all fats are unhealthy. Polyunsaturated fats and monounsaturated fats are the healthier fats compared to saturated fats. Some of these fats are high in anti-inflammatory properties and have a rich source of Vitamin E. Foods that contain unsaturated fats include; nuts, seeds, avocados, olive oil, soybean oil, canola oil, avocado oil, peanut oil and vegetable oil. It is important to understand that these fats are still high in calories - therefore, portions should be monitored. These fats, however, are preferred over saturated fats.

Saturated fats, on the other hand, can increase inflammation. Some examples of saturated fats are high fat dairy foods (whole milk, half and half, cheeses, butter, and ice cream), fried foods, commercial baked goods, creamed vegetables/soups/sauces, sausages, Italian meats, red meat, animal fat, and processed meat products.

Low Calorie Foods: Avoid drenching your food in dressing, oil, butter, and sugar, which can increase your calorie intake. High calorie foods can cause weight gain and inflammation so it is important to make healthy choices when choosing what foods to eat.

Antioxidants: It remains unproven whether diets high in antioxidants can help with inflammation associated with lupus. Fruits and vegetables are sources of antioxidants such as Vitamin A, Vitamin C, Vitamin E, Selenium, Carotenes, and Bioflavonoids.

High Calcium and Vitamin D Intake: Foods high in calcium and vitamin D promote healthy bones. Some medications for lupus deplete your body of calcium, so including calcium in your diet is essential. It can be found in foods like wild salmon (with bones), enriched/fortified soy milk, mushrooms (shitake), broccoli, kale, sardines (with bones), fortified milk, and fortified breakfast cereals. The recommendation for calcium intake is slightly different for men and women. For women less than 50 years of age, the recommendation is 1000 mg. For women over 50 years of age, the recommendation is 1200 mg. For men ages 50 to 70, the recommendation is 1000 mg and for those older than 70 years of age, it is 1200 mg. Vitamin D recommendation is the same for both men and women. For people less than 70 years of age, the recommendation is 600 IU a day and for those over 70 years of age, the recommendation is 800 IU a day.

Grains: Grains are a good source of fiber and energy, foliate, B6, B2, selenium, and zinc, and are naturally low in fat. Some whole grain foods include brown and wild rice, whole wheat bread, whole wheat pasta, rye, oats, quinoa, corn, and barley.

Dairy: Dairy products hold the richest source of calcium and provide a good amount of protein, vitamin D, selenium, B vitamins, and zinc. Foods high in calcium are shown to help build strong teeth and bones, which are very important for lupus patients because of their high risk of osteoporosis.

When choosing dairy products, remember to go either low-fat or fat-free. Some examples include 1% and skim milk, low fat and low sodium yogurt, and low fat cheese. Foods to avoid are 2% and whole milk, which contain a large amount of fat and cholesterol. If you do not or cannot consume milk, choose lactose-free milk, soy milk, and almond milk that are fortified with calcium and Vitamin D. Aim for three or more servings a day.

Meat, Fish, and Poultry: They contain zinc and B vitamins and are a good source of Omega-3 fatty acids and protein to maintain muscle. Here are some healthy tips when buying and preparing your meats, fish, and poultry:

- Red meat is high in cholesterol and saturated fat. Try to limit it to once a week if you can.
- Look for lean meats around 99%.
- Remove skin from poultry because that is where the most saturated fat is.
- Trim any visible fat off when preparing meat.

- Broil and grill vs. pan fried with oil, deep fried, and breading.

- It is important to incorporate fish into your diet around 3-4 times a week.

- Practice portion control - meat should not take up ½ of your plate, it should be more like ¼

- Best Bets: chicken breast, turkey breast, lean pork, wild salmon, herring, mackerel, sardines, anchovies, rainbow trout, tuna (canned light in water), crab, oysters, tilapia, cod.

Omega 3 Fatty Acids: Research indicates that omega 3 fatty acids from fish or fish oils may help manage high triglycerides and heart disease. Foods rich in omega 3 fatty acids include salmon, sardines, mackerel, bluefish, herring, mullet, tuna, halibut, lake trout, rainbow trout, ground flaxseed, chia seeds, walnuts, pecans, canola oil, walnut oil, and flaxseed oil, and are part of a heart-healthy meal plan.

Tips to incorporate Omega 3's into your diet:
- Add chopped nuts to salads
- Add grilled salmon, tuna, and sardines to salad
- Snack on nuts
- Sprinkle ground flaxseeds on cereal and yogurt

Beans, Nuts, and Seeds: Good source of vitamin E, selenium, protein, and fiber. Some foods that you can snack on throughout the day include:
- Brazil nuts
- Wheat germ
- Flaxseed

- Chia seeds

- Soybeans

- Kidney beans

- Tofu

- Walnuts

- Lentils

When purchasing, look for beans that are unsalted and low in sodium. When buying canned beans, make sure to rinse and drain excess liquid to remove extra sodium.

What Foods Should You Avoid?

- Foods high in saturated fat, trans fat, and cholesterol

- Red meats and high fat meats like liver, organ meats, and dark meats.

- Alcoholic beverages, salty foods, sweetened beverages, candy, snacks, sweets, and alfalfa sprouts.
- These foods can worsen side effects of steroids: Simple carbohydrates and refined carbohydrates (often processed)
- Overly processed foods:
    - ☐ Processed foods often have added salt and sugar, so try and eat fresh.
    - ☐ When foods are processed that means that modifications have been made to the product where fiber or vitamins were removed
    - ☐ Know that if a food or beverage has a food label it has been processed, so be aware of what is in it.

4.2 Exercise and Physical Activity

If you're living with lupus, regular physical activity can be an important part of your overall treatment plan. Staying active can boost your energy levels, improve joint flexibility, and help alleviate stress.

Before you begin an exercise routine, talk with your healthcare professional to get the go-ahead and determine the best plan for your needs.

To minimize stress on your joints and muscles, opt for activities such as walking, cycling, and swimming. Gentle yoga, Pilates, and cardio workouts are also excellent options.

Be consistent with your workout routine and include a diverse range of exercises that target all major muscle groups. Continuously challenging your body with different movements and activities can help keep your workouts engaging.

Go at your own pace and work within your limits. If your workouts cause stress or overwhelm you for any reason, including a packed schedule, reduce the intensity or duration of your routines. Allow yourself ample time to rest and recover.

Sample Lupus Workout Routine

Tree Pose: This pose focuses on balance, strength, and stability. It also encourages relaxation, helps still your mind, and may restore a sense of inner calmness.

- From standing, shift your weight onto your left foot.
- Slowly lift your right foot off the floor.

- Rotate the sole of your right foot to face the inner part of your left leg.
- Place your foot on your outer ankle, calf, or thigh. Avoid placing your foot directly on your knee.
- Place your hands in any comfortable position.
- Hold this position for up to 1 minute.
- Repeat on the opposite side.

Squats: This exercise improves stability and core strength while targeting your glutes, quadriceps, and hamstrings to develop lower body strength.

- Stand with feet hip distance apart or slightly wider.
- Raise your arms to shoulder level in front of your body.

- Bend your knees to lower yourself into a squat position.
- Pause for a moment before returning to the starting position.
- Do 1–3 sets of 8–12 repetitions.

High Lunges: Lunges are an excellent exercise to improve strength, balance, and stability.

- Stand with your feet hip-width apart.
- Step your left foot forward, aligning your knee directly above or slightly behind your ankle.
- Bend both knees until your back knee is just above the floor.
- Lengthen your spine and engage your core for stability.
- Push through your front heel to return to the starting position.

- Repeat on the opposite side.
- Do 1–3 sets of 8-12 repetitions.

Plank: This exercise strengthens your shoulders, core, and hamstrings. It also improves joint stability.

- Begin on all fours, with your hands directly under your shoulders.
- Straighten your legs and lift your heels, raising your hips to align your spine.
- Activate your abdominal, arm, and leg muscles to create stability.
- Lengthen the back of your neck and release any tension in your shoulders.
- Hold this position for up to 1 minute.
- Repeat 1–3 times.Bridge pose

Bridge Pose: This exercise targets your cores, glutes, and hamstrings. For optimal alignment, place a small ball, cushion, or yoga block between your knees.

- Lie on your back with your knees bent and your feet pressing firmly into the floor.
- Slowly lift your hips off the floor.
- Hold this position for 5 breaths.
- Lower your hips to the starting position.
- Do 1–3 sets of 8–12 repetitions.

4.3 Importance of Sleep and Stress Management

Adequate and quality sleep plays a significant role in managing Lupus symptoms. However, the condition itself, along with associated factors, can often lead to sleep disturbances. Here's why sleep is crucial:

- Symptom Management: Quality sleep helps in managing symptoms like fatigue, joint pain, and cognitive function often experienced by individuals with Lupus.

- Immune Function: Sleep is vital for immune system function, and inadequate sleep may further weaken an already compromised immune system in Lupus.

- Reduced Inflammation: Quality sleep contributes to reducing inflammation, which is a hallmark feature of Lupus.

Managing stress is equally important, as stress can potentially trigger or exacerbate Lupus symptoms. Here's why stress management is crucial:

- Flare Prevention: Stressful situations can lead to flares or worsening of symptoms in individuals with Lupus.

- Impact on Immune System: Stress can weaken the immune system, making it harder for the body to manage inflammation and fight infections.

- Quality of Life: Effective stress management techniques can significantly improve the overall quality of life for individuals with Lupus.

Strategies for Sleep and Stress Management

Establishing Sleep Hygiene: Creating a sleep-friendly environment, maintaining a regular sleep schedule, and adopting relaxation techniques before bedtime can promote better sleep.

Physical Activity: Engaging in gentle exercises or activities suited to individual abilities can improve sleep quality and reduce stress levels.

Mindfulness and Relaxation: Practices like meditation, deep breathing exercises, or yoga can effectively reduce stress and promote relaxation.

Limiting Stimulants: Avoiding caffeine, nicotine, and electronic devices before bedtime can aid in better sleep quality.

Setting Boundaries: Establishing boundaries, prioritizing tasks, and seeking support in managing responsibilities can reduce stress levels.

Professional Help: Seeking guidance from healthcare providers or counselors specialized in stress management techniques can provide valuable strategies.

Self-Care Practices: Engaging in activities that bring joy and relaxation, such as hobbies, reading, or spending time in nature, contributes to stress reduction.

Chapter 5: Lupus and Relationship

5.1 Navigating Relationships with Families and Friends

Whether you consider your family as the family you were born or married into, the one you've created with your partner or spouse, or one you've hand-picked from close friends over the years, the strong support system these people provide in your life is as vital to your health and well-being as any medication that may be prescribed to treat your lupus.

Your kids may run to you as the one who helps them with their homework. Your partner or spouse may rely on you to do the grocery shopping, fix the car or clean the house. Your friends may expect you to plan road trips or nights on the town. With a lupus diagnosis, however, those roles and expectations may have to change to some degree. The question is, how to take this opportunity – create healthy, new expectations for whatever changes need to occur in your relationships and even make them stronger?

First and foremost, it's important to try to not feel guilty about changes in your role as a member of the family. You have to take care of yourself and make yourself a priority – maybe for the first time in your life – in order to, in turn, be there for others. Second, you may have to change how you communicate with your loved ones in order to be heard and ensure needs are met – developing assertiveness skills is a boon. Third, you need to get comfortable telling others exactly how you are feeling and asking for help – you may have to ask your spouse or partner to pick up dinner, your kids to do their own laundry, or your friends to drive you to an event. This will undoubtedly be awkward at first, but in time you'll develop a routine and it should become second nature and the "new norm" for all involved.

5.2 Lupus in the Workplace

Managing lupus while working full time (or even part time) can be tricky, especially when you can't predict when you'll have symptoms or how bad they'll be. Changes to your work schedule and environment can help you stay productive. So can strategies to deal with your symptoms.

You may or may not decide to tell your boss and co-workers about your condition. But if you do, federal disability laws require your employer to give you reasonable accommodations to help you do your job. Lupus symptoms like brain fog, fatigue, and pain can get in the way of your workload. To minimize them, first work with your doctor to come up with an effective treatment plan.

Beyond that, try these tricks to manage brain fog on the job:

Minimize Distractions and Avoid Multitasking: Concentrating on one thing at a time makes it easier to focus. You might pause emails when you're working on a project. Or wear noise-canceling headphones at times when you don't need to interact with customers or co-workers.

Pace Yourself: Allow extra time when you're working on something that requires concentration. It helps to plan out multi-step projects in writing. Let your boss or co-workers know if you need help.

Visual Cues Can Help: If you often forget things, leave yourself visual reminders. For example, put your headset on your keyboard to remind yourself about a recording you need to transcribe.

Fatigue is one of the most common symptoms that affects people with lupus. To deal with fatigue on the job, you might:

Prioritize: Plan your work schedule ahead of time, if you can. Highlight the most important tasks so you can focus on them first. If you tend to get tired at certain times of day, schedule high-priority tasks for times when you have the most energy.

Don't Skimp on Rest: A good night's sleep helps you start the day with as much energy as possible. Schedule breaks throughout your day, if possible.

Change Your Environment or Hours: Ask your boss if you can telework on days you're feeling especially fatigued. If you usually stand up to do your job, see if you can sit for at least part of the time. A flexible schedule might help if you have less energy at certain times of day.

Enlist Help: Think about tasks you can delegate so you can focus on critical tasks that require your attention. And don't underestimate the value of a good support network at home. That gives you more time to relax so you go to work well-rested.

It's hard to concentrate on work when you're in pain. Talk to your doctor about pain management. And take sick days when you need them. Some other things to try include:

Helpful Equipment: A more comfortable chair can make a difference. If typing hurts your fingers, try voice-to-text technology. A mobility scooter might be an option if you do lots of walking on the job.

Movement Breaks: Even a little exercise can reduce pain. Build several movement breaks into your day. Don't sit in one position for long stretches.

Hot or Cold Therapy: Some people get pain relief from heating pads. Others find that an ice pack helps. Try keeping one of these on hand at your workplace.

5.3 Support Systems and Building a Support Network

Whether you have lupus or are a caregiver to someone with lupus, a strong support network is critical to maintaining optimal health and keeping the normal stresses of life in check. Just as it takes a medical team to manage lupus, living well with lupus requires a team of people who offer support — emotional, physical and spiritual. There are steps to help you build and grow your social support network. Once your network is in place, you'll find it to be invaluable day to day and through the years.

Know the Dangers of Isolation: It's easy to be overwhelmed when you're managing a chronic disease like lupus, or when caring for someone else. This is when it's most important to reach out to your support network. The dangers of isolation may start small, but a lack of interaction with others can negatively affect your health and well-being over time. Spending time alone is not the same as being isolated. Alone time is sometimes a good thing. Being isolated, however, is not.

A chronic illness like lupus can be isolating for many reasons. You can become isolated if you don't understand or know anyone else who has the disease. You can also feel isolated if you have always been healthy until lupus developed. This can affect your social life, work or even school.

Being assured that you are a valuable member of society and that you matter to the people in your life will help you feel more secure. Using daily positive affirmations can help, too.

Reach Out: Research shows that getting the help you need (known as "perceived social support") improves your quality of life, whether you have lupus or you're a caregiver. A strong support team will have people who can help in different ways. However, it's not necessary, or likely, that everyone in your support network can meet all of your needs. The important thing is that you can count on these people when you need them.

The individuals who make up your support network can include:

- Family members: A lupus diagnosis affects the whole family. You may find that cousins, aunts, uncles, siblings and your spouse will empathize and naturally step up into the role of supporter.

- Neighbors: People in your neighborhood often can provide a home-cooked meal during a stressful time, or they can simply be a nearby source of comfort.

- Coworkers: The people you work with can help by being empathetic about your situation. You may need to telecommute, take a leave of absence or use flex time, which will require the cooperation and support of your colleagues.

- Lupus Support Group Members: People in this network have knowledge about lupus and can offer strategies and suggestions based on their experience.

- Medical Team: If you're a caregiver, your loved one's providers and office staff, social workers, and other professionals will probably understand what you are going through and can be supportive of your caregiving role.

- Therapist or Counselor: It's important that you have an outlet for your emotions. Check to see if mental health services are included in your employer's health coverage. If not, look for free services in your community.

- Teachers and School Instructors: When you are caring for a child with lupus, keep his or her teachers informed and let them know how they can help.

Set Up Several Types of Support: The first part of putting together your support network is really identifying what you need. Define what you think will fill that void, and explore all the different opportunities that may be available. Know the different types of support to rely on:

- emotional support
- physical and mental wellness
- task related support
- support groups
- spiritual support
- family support

Ask: By asking for help, it may feel like you are giving up your independence, but most people want to help. Although they may not completely understand what you're going through, they want to be supportive. It is important to understand how to make your needs known to people who can assist you. Learning to ask for help, and learning to accept help that is offered, will get easier over time. Not everybody has the skills to seek out support, especially if you're a little socially shy. If it feels awkward to make a request, it may require practice initiating certain conversations. Knowing what you need help with, and having a list of people you think would be good matches for those roles, will make each 'ask' much easier. Next to people's names, put their strengths: what they like to do and what they do well.

Connect: You can get started by connecting with communities online launched by the Lupus

Foundation of America that provides people with lupus and their loved ones a safe and understanding space to share experiences, find emotional support, and discuss ways to manage the disease.

Share: You'll probably find that you share different aspects of what you're going through with different people. That's why it's so helpful to have a variety of people to talk with and places where you can speak and be heard. People's emotions are very complicated when they're dealing with chronic illness. Regular meetings with an objective person, such as a trained counselor or therapist, can be very helpful. You may also want to engage with people who understand lupus and know what you're going through.

Volunteer: Volunteerism offers social support benefits because helping others can make you feel better about life in general. One good option is volunteering for a Lupus Foundation of America chapter or a support group.

Think about the social causes you are passionate about and the skills you have to offer. Check out an organization's website for volunteer opportunities, or call the local office and ask how you can help.

Chapter 6: Advocacy and Wellness

6.1 Spreading Lupus Awareness

Lupus is often misunderstood, and raising awareness is essential to dispel myths, reduce stigma, and garner support. Increased awareness contributes to:

- Early Diagnosis: Improved awareness can lead to earlier detection and diagnosis of Lupus, facilitating better disease management.

- Support Systems: Enhanced awareness fosters supportive environments within communities, families, and workplaces.

- Research Funding: Increased public knowledge can generate interest and support for Lupus research, potentially leading to advancements in treatment and understanding.

Effective Advocacy Strategies

Education Campaigns:

- Online Platforms: Utilize social media, blogs, and websites to share educational content about Lupus, including its symptoms, treatment options, and the daily challenges faced by those living with the condition.
- Infographics and Visuals: Create visually appealing content that simplifies complex information about Lupus for easy understanding and sharing.

Community Events:

- Local Workshops and Seminars: Organize or participate in local events to educate communities about Lupus. Collaborate with healthcare professionals, support groups, and local organizations to maximize impact.

- Health Fairs: Participate in health fairs to provide informational pamphlets, conduct brief awareness sessions, and engage with the community.

Collaboration with Advocacy Organizations:

- Partnering with Nonprofits: Collaborate with Lupus-focused nonprofit organizations to amplify awareness efforts. Leverage their resources, networks, and campaigns to reach a broader audience.

- Advocacy Days: Participate in or organize advocacy days to connect with policymakers, urging them to prioritize Lupus research and support.

Media Engagement:

- Press Releases: Share press releases about Lupus awareness events, new research findings, or personal stories to garner media attention.
- Interviews and Features: Seek opportunities for interviews or features in local newspapers, magazines, radio shows, or podcasts to share insights about Lupus.

Awareness Merchandise:

- Branded Merchandise: Create and distribute branded Lupus awareness merchandise, such as T-shirts, wristbands, or pins, to generate interest and visibility.

- Online Stores: Set up online stores selling awareness merchandise, with proceeds directed toward Lupus research or support programs.

Storytelling and Personal Experiences:

- Blogs and Personal Stories: Encourage individuals living with Lupus to share their stories through blogs, articles, or personal testimonies to humanize the experience and create relatable narratives.
- Social Media Campaigns: Launch campaigns encouraging individuals to share their Lupus journeys using specific hashtags to create a collective voice.

6.2 Advocacy Efforts and Initiatives

Advocacy involves speaking up, influencing decisions, and promoting change. In the context of Lupus, advocacy aims to:

Raise Awareness: Educate the public, policymakers, and healthcare professionals about Lupus, its impact, and the needs of those affected.

Improve Access to Care: Advocate for better access to quality healthcare, treatment options, and support services for individuals with Lupus.

Advance Research and Funding: Push for increased funding and support for Lupus research to develop better treatments and ultimately find a cure.

Effective Advocacy Strategies

Policy Advocacy

- Legislative Outreach: Engage policymakers and legislators to advocate for policies that support individuals with Lupus, such as improved healthcare coverage or funding for research programs.
- Legislative Calls to Action: Encourage supporters to contact their representatives to advocate for Lupus-related legislation or policies.

Community Engagement:

- Awareness Campaigns: Organize community-based awareness campaigns, walks, or events to educate and engage the public in Lupus advocacy efforts.

- Support Group Advocacy: Collaborate with local support groups to advocate collectively for community needs and resources.

Collaboration with Organizations:

- Partnerships with Advocacy Groups: Partner with national or local advocacy organizations focused on Lupus to amplify advocacy efforts and leverage resources.
- Coalition Building: Form coalitions with other disease-specific advocacy groups to advocate for common interests, share resources, and strengthen advocacy efforts.

Media and Public Relations:

- Public Awareness Campaigns: Use various media platforms to disseminate information, personal stories, and calls to action for Lupus awareness and advocacy.
- Media Outreach: Collaborate with journalists, bloggers, and influencers to highlight Lupus-related issues and stories.

Education and Training:

- Training Sessions: Conduct training sessions or workshops to equip advocates with the knowledge and skills needed to effectively advocate for Lupus-related causes.
- Educational Materials: Develop educational resources and toolkits to empower advocates and the public with accurate information about Lupus.

Chapter 7: Empowering Stories

Katherine's Story

"I got diagnosed with Lupus, late December 2014. By the time I was diagnosed, it was about four months into my first proper flare, and I couldn't lift myself to sit, let alone walk. I was in such pain I didn't think I was able to bear; I'd scream out "MY BRAIN IS ON FIRE!" because it usually felt like that. And I begged to have my toes cut off because it felt like someone held a candle to my feet. It's difficult to understand if you haven't experienced it. That's one of the reasons I try to raise awareness about this cruel disease that ravages you from the inside without cause. I was 24 when I got diagnosed, but since I was 5, Lupus had been terrorizing me with various symptoms, the most dreadful: Rheumatoid Arthritis. I cannot accurately describe how terrible it was to always have to carry balms and painkillers on my person and to fear cold weather. Now, I have more than painkillers, and probably should invest in my local pharmacies, lol, but I live a life constantly filled with gratitude. I try not to take anything for granted and I appreciate anyone who shows the slightest interest in learning about this condition that scarred me in so many ways, and physically too. Sometimes I catch people staring at me and it usually takes about 2 seconds to remember I have no hair on my head, and I smile at their curiosity. Then I giggle to myself because I think "Bet you wouldn't imagine anything like Lupus did this." But Lupus did and still does take my hair, so I chopped it all off because I refuse to be at its mercy. Life is much slower for me now and that's a good thing. I keep learning to differentiate what's important from everything drawing my attention; I cannot afford any form of stress. Some days are tougher than others, but every day, I remind myself I'm not only a warrior because of the battle I fight, I'm also a victor because I win".

Mary's Story

"Up until my diagnosis, I had a clean bill of health. I spent six months in 2016 visiting different hospitals just to get answers to why I suddenly felt my body had decided to go rogue on me. In those six months, my symptoms were fatigue, fever, loss of appetite and unexplainable hunger (which was just confusing – one minute I didn't feel like eating, the next I felt like eating a house). I also experienced muscle aches (these were constant all through and I still have them now), ulcers of the mouth and morning stiffness (wherein the first fifteen minutes of the day I wouldn't be able to move any part of my body. So I just lay there like a log of wood waiting for the stiffness to subside). There were occasional facial rashes; also known as the butterfly rashes – red rashes all over my face. I just woke up and saw those rashes sometimes. And whenever I had them, I found it difficult to step out of my room. Then there were chest pains, numbness in fingers and feet and heat stroke. I usually experienced heat stroke, which made my knees buckle and left me struggling to breathe. And how can I forget the excruciating pains in my joints and the hair loss? At first, I thought it was my hair breaking; so I cut it often, only to still have it fall off, leaving bald spots. Since my diagnosis, I have struggled not only physically but also emotionally. I felt shutting everyone out made sense. Now I have a group of women who understand me, who share my fears and worries but also push me to be better. They all say starting the foundation has helped them but they have healed me, Their collective strength blows me away. This lupus will not define us or cripple us".

Sarah's Story

"I'm 28 years old. I was diagnosed with lupus erythematosus in February of 2015. It has since progressed to affecting the tissues of my kidneys, eyes, and heart. I've also been diagnosed with peripheral neuropathy, CKD(chronic kidney disease), hypertensive heart disease and fibromyalgia. It was an excruciatingly painful, miserable and difficult illness to navigate but, I've come to terms with the condition and have also made lifestyle changes to make the journey easier for me. I have also been able to educate my family and loved ones about the condition so that they don't get extremely worried when I experience a flare-up. I have been able to continue with my career as an entrepreneur and to the best of my ability I've managed my daily routines as well. I know that lupus can't beat me and I'm eternally grateful for the support I've gotten from my fellow warriors"

Chapter 8: Future Prospects in Lupus Research

There is much hope on the horizon for people with lupus, as researchers are making strides in better understanding the disease and developing new treatments. For example, researchers are exploring the role of genetics in lupus and how certain genes may play a role in triggering the disease. They are also investigating new ways to target the immune system to reduce inflammation and improve outcomes for people with lupus. Additionally, there is ongoing research into potential biomarkers that could help diagnose lupus earlier and more accurately. There is also hope for better treatments that can target the specific symptoms that each person experiences.

In addition to the research currently underway, there are also many new clinical trials being conducted to test new treatments for lupus. For example, researchers are testing new medications that target specific immune pathways involved in the disease. They are also investigating the use of stem cell therapy and gene therapy to treat lupus. These new therapies have the potential to significantly improve outcomes for people with lupus. As these treatments are being studied, researchers are also working to understand how to prevent lupus from developing in the first place.

If you're reading this book, Lupus Awareness, you may also be interested in my books on osteoporosis and heart disease. Tap the links to read them.

Thank you for purchasing my book. I'd really appreciate it if you could take a moment to leave a review. Your feedback will help me improve and make my next book even better. I'm always looking forward to improving, so please do not hold back! Thank you for your time and support.